SADHANA

IN

SRI AUROBINDO'S YOGA

M. P. PANDIT

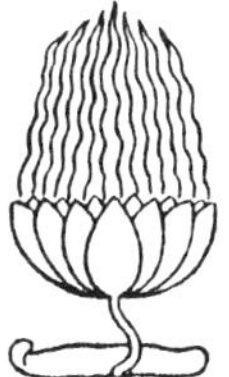

Publisher:

Auromere, a department of
Atmaniketan Ashram Inc.

TO THE **MOTHER**

WHO HAS OPENED

THE DOORS OF

THE AGE OF GOLD.

Contents:

Introduction

THE immense range of the prolific pen of Sri Aurobindo is matched only by the Olympian quality of the writing that flows from it. He wrote his first poem in his eleventh year ; his last writing, 'The Mind of Light', in his seventy-eighth. The subjects that received the alchemic touch of this divine man are varied : Art, Poetry, Criticism, Philosophy, Religion, Sociology, Polity, History, Yoga—all these are treated with a depth of insight and universality of outlook which bring to the fore their meeting ground in a commonness of purpose. Whatever the period, earlier or later, whatever the subject, the spirit that governs all his writings is the Ideal of Perfection of Man, the Gospel of Divine Life on earth. Whether it is the romantic dramas of the early years of his literary activity or the pungent editorials and fiery utterances during the political phase of his meteoric career or it is the metaphysics of his Teaching, the keynote of his writing is always the same—the divine potentiality of man.

And indeed, it could not be otherwise. For, the Truth he came to fulfil, the Ideal for which he devoted the major part of his life on earth is the possibility, nay, the inevitability, of a New Life for the human race. This consummation of the æonic labour of Nature in evolution is sought to be effected by a revolutionary precipitation of its process by which a new Consciousness shall manifest and impel the life on earth, bringing about a radical change in its character; in a word, deliver human life from the hold of Ignorance, Incapacity and Death into the freedom of a divine Knowledge, Power and Immortality.

Sri Aurobindo develops this theme and expounds it in all the ramifications of a metaphysical system in his basic work, 'The Life Divine'. The means for translating this Doctrine into practice and the experience which gives life to the theory, is described in his other great work, 'The Synthesis of Yoga'. How this urge in man for a total self-perfection is reflected in the development of society and how this ideal of self-fulfilment can be worked out in collectivity is shown in 'The Human Cycle'. 'The Ideal of Human Unity' traces the lines on which the far spread peoples of the globe are slowly but steadily moving towards an overt realisation of the Truth of Oneness that is governing their development from within, analyses the nature of the obstructions delaying the achievement and indicates the direction in which the solution is to be found.

Sri Aurobindo then proceeds to see how far this Knowledge of his perception and experience is consistent with the main spiritual and cultural tradition of India and for this purpose takes up the ancient texts of her Scriptures. He goes straight to the core of the hymns of the Rig Veda, bares the thought-structure that is embedded in them and gathers in a methodical form the various hints scattered all over these remnants of a rich hymnal past, signposts of the inner discipline perfected by the Rishis for their self-culture and development. His findings are set forth in the series on the 'Secret of the Veda' and in his translations of a large number of hymns and commentaries on them, now collected together under two titles, 'On the Veda' and 'Hymns to the Mystic Fire'.

Similarly with the Upanishads. He translates and gives a detailed exposition of the thought in the Isha and Kena Upanishads[1] drawing attention to the comprehensive character of their teaching which embraces the whole world as a purposeful manifestation of the all-pervading Brahman, Brahman that is Knowledge-Power-Bliss. He has besides given free renderings of the Katha, Prashna, Taittiriya, Aitareya, Mundaka and Mandukya texts[2] and annotated upon certain key concepts in the Taittiriya, the Chhandogya[3] and the Brihadaranyaka.[4]

Next, he takes the Gita which records a high watermark reached by the turn for synthesis characteristic of the Indian genius. He expounds with a convincing thoroughness the manifold Way prescribed in it for the application of the gains of the Spirit to the dynamic side of life—activity—as also for the use of action for the growth of the being Godward. These brilliant 'Essays on the Gita' are among the most widely read of his writings.

In all these studies, be it noted, Sri Aurobindo does not rely on any of the extant commentaries for arriving at the import of the scriptures. His is a straightforward approach of an open mind and his conclusions are seen to be well tested on internal and circumstantial evidence of the texts themselves.

Besides these major sequences in his writings which we have dwelt upon elsewhere,[5] there is a large number of works,[6] smaller in bulk but not less significant for that reason. We propose to study some of these works, notably those which have an important bearing on the practical side, the Sadhana, of the Teaching of Sri Aurobindo.

And of them, naturally, first comes 'THE MOTHER '.

NOTES ON INTRODUCTION

[1] *Isha Upanishad, Kena Upanishad.*
[2] *Eight Upanishads.*
[3] Vide *Advent*, Vol. X, No. 3.
[4] *Sri Aurobindo Mandir Annual* No. 12.
[5] *The Teaching of Sri Aurobindo.*
[6] There is a considerable mass of poetry by Sri Aurobindo in English the most important of which is the Epic, *Savitri: A legend and a symbol,* in which he sketches the whole gamut of the spiritual adventure of humanity and embodies in it the course, the scope and achievement of his own mission for the transfiguration of mortal life into a Poem of Immortality. But this is a vast subject by itself and falls outside the limits we have set for ourselves here.

The Mother

THOUGH slender in volume, this work occupies a key position in the Yoga literature of Sri Aurobindo. For, it lays down in detail the steps of the Sadhana, the indispensable discipline that is to be practised if one is to realise the object of this Yoga which is nothing less than the transformation of human life into a divine living.

The task is formidable, indeed, impossible to achieve by human effort alone. It is only the Divine Shakti at work in the universe, in the Creation projected by Herself and led by Herself for the fulfilment of Her own Purpose, that can accomplish it. She is to be invoked and in Her hands placed the sadhana. But there are conditions in which alone the Supreme Shakti will act.

There must be, in the first place, an *aspiration* in you for the higher Truth. It is not enough that the aspiration is there ; it must be intense, it must pervade more and more all the parts of your being so that the whole is afire with a live incessant call for the Divine Power to manifest itself.

Consistent with this dynamic aspiration you have to learn to *surrender* yourself to the Higher

Shakti. You must gather up all your movements and deliver yourself to the Power with a complete submission to its Will and command. The surrender must be active, cooperative, not tamasic and inert. There must be besides an exclusive self-opening to the Divine working and to no other. It defeats your purpose if you invoke the Divine Power and at the same time allow in you movements that are alien to the Truth of your seeking. At every step there has to be a *rejection* of all that proceeds from what is not the Truth, not the Light. The rejection has to be entire. There should be no acceptance or even sympathy anywhere in you with any element of falsehood and ignorance.

This triple labour of aspiration, rejection and surrender is the contribution demanded of you. For although it is true that it is the Divine Shakti who really carries out the sadhana in you, yet so long as you remain subject to the lower nature your personal effort is indispensable; you have to exert to overcome this nature. And in proportion as you rise above it and place yourself in the charge of the Higher Power, your effort is gradually replaced by the working of the Shakti. And there is no limit to the wonders that the Shakti, the Divine Grace, can effect in you. Only, from your side is asked a constant faith, sincerity and utter surrender. The more complete they are, the more secure the protection and sure the progress.

The ideal sadhaka is one who is conscious of

the Divine not only in himself but everywhere. All is Divine in origin and all has to be won back for the Divine, releasing it from the hold of the lords of Ignorance and Falsehood. Of the forces and powers put out from the Divine, the most usurped and the most misused are the forces of Wealth, Power and Sex. The seeker of the Integral Path has not to renounce but to exert and reconquer them, yoke them to the Purpose of the Divine. And this he can do only if he is free from the taint of desire and attachment, attains an equality of mind and purity of heart.

To be a true worker of the Divine, one needs to be totally free from desire and ego, the twin mainsprings of normal human activity. A perfect doer of Divine Works is one who is perfectly identified with the Divine Consciousness. But such an identification can only come as a culmination of a self-giving process. In the beginning of this sadhana, the sadhaka does the work that is given him as work for the Divine Mother. He seeks no personal gain. To do service to Her, to offer works to Her is its own reward. Her pleasure is his fulfilment. In time the sense of his being a worker gradually recedes and the consciousness of an instrument replaces it. His increasing devotion for the Mother brings about such an inner contact and intimacy that he has only to refer things to Her and he receives Her instant guidance. Not only guidance, but also the force to effectuate it. The sadhaka begins to realise that all powers and faculties are only channels for Her Force and action. And as this closeness and identification with the Mother increase in their pervasion and intensity, the sadhaka feels no longer a worker or a servant or an instrument. He feels and realises in his being, that he is a child of Hers, truly a part of Her Consciousness. All his movements are consciously felt to be Her Movements. He is just a mould of Her Knowledge, Her Force, Her Ananda.

Who is the Divine Mother to whom the seeker is called upon to make a complete surrender and who carries him safe in Her arms through the perilous path? How is She felt and seen? How does She work and pour Herself in the human vessel? Sri Aurobindo reveals this Knowledge in the last and the major part of the work which is aptly described as the *Mātṛ Upaniṣad*. Here in one matchless prose-poem winging out of his luminous Seer-Vision, he lays bare the secret lore of the Manifestation of the Divine Mother for the liberation and perfection of man and the revelation of the Supreme on earth.

*   *   *

The Consciousness-Force of the One Supreme Being is the Mother of all creation. For it is this Divine Conscious Force, Shakti, that brings the worlds into manifestation out of the Being, upbears and leads them in their career, in a word, mothers them. There are three ways of Her being in which it is possible to be aware of Her. She has three statuses.

Transcendent, She is above all the worlds, linking the Supreme Being to all creation. She it is who bears the Supreme in Her consciousness, calls and holds the truths to be manifested and casts them into form. All is Her Lila with the Lord.

Universal, She spreads Herself out as the substance and the soul of each universe of Her creation. It is Her presence that gives life and meaning to all, Her movement that gives the direction.

Individual, She embodies in Herself both the transcendent and the universal ways of Her existence and makes their Power operative here for the manifestation of the Divine in each individual form. She descends in person into the world of Ignorance in order to uplift and release it from the Falsehood and obscurity into which it has sunk.

The Divine Mother has many aspects, many personalities, that severally express the plenitude of Her oceanic Being. Of these, Sri Aurobindo points to the Four which have most to do with and are incessantly active for the evolution of this universe towards its destined goal of Perfection in the verities of Knowledge, Power and Ananda. They are Maheshwari, Mahakali, Mahalakshmi and Mahasaraswati.

Maheshwari is the Personality who presides over the infinite expanses of Knowledge. She builds the human soul and nature into the Divine Truth and opens out our summits into the splendours of the supreme Light.

Mahakali embodies an all-effectuating Power and Will. Hers is the divine Warrior-Force that smashes all obstruction and speeds upward human aspiration and effort.

Mahalakshmi is the soul of all Beauty and Harmony in creation. It is She who manifests the hidden Bliss in life and prepares the receptacles for the divine Ananda.

Mahasaraswati holds in Herself an inexhaustible capacity for flawless work and exact perfection. Nearest of the Four to physical Nature, She is most concerned with organisation, execution and construction, all of which She carries out with a thoroughness that is integral.

Sri Aurobindo's narration of the characteristics of these Four Powers of the Divine Mother, their ways of working, their conditions to manifest, their mission of love and labour for man, forms one of the most enthralling pieces of the spiritual literature of all time.

There are other Powers too of the Divine Mother. But they are more in the background and will manifest only when these Four have established and founded their harmony. Then will their supramental action be possible which alone can finally deliver the thrice bound nature into the dynamic freedom of the Spirit.

If you seek this transformation, be surrendered absolutely in the hands of the Divine Mother; be always conscious in every part of your being,—mind, soul, life, the very cells of the body-consciousness—of the presence of the Mother and the workings of Her Powers; and be plastic to Her touch, ever pliant to comply with the demands of Her Force, to be shaped at all moments and in all movements in the mould of Her choice. For only so can the supreme Truth, Light and Ananda be brought down into this world of falsehood, obscurity and suffering, and human nature transmuted into a divine supernature.

The Yoga and its Objects

THERE are yogas and yogas. Each yoga has its own means; some base themselves on the physical organism, some on the life-dynamism, some on the emotional, others on the mental faculties, and yet others seek to combine in their method one means with another. But all of them, broadly speaking, have one aim viz. to heighten the state of one's being above and beyond the normal bounds of the body and life and attain a release into a freedom of self-existence or non-existence—*mukti*. The yoga of which Sri Aurobindo speaks here, however, is of a different kind. It is distinctive in its aim and distinctive also in its means. The object of this Yoga is not liberation, *mukti*, but fulfilment, *sampatti*. Fulfilment of what? of the Will of God in Creation. And what is that Will?

The Divine has projected the universe out of His own Being with a purpose. That purpose is to manifest Himself, His inalienable nature of Existence, Consciousness and Bliss, *saccidānanda*. It is the aim of our Yoga to work out this Supreme Will by the liberation of human life from the holds of Ignorance, Limitation and Death and its transformation into the divine nature of Knowledge, Infinity and Immortality. The whole of man,—not the mind alone, or the soul alone,—is to be taken up and subjected to the transforming change. All the faculties of the being are to be yoked to this One Purpose. This is the means, and this the goal of our Yoga which is indeed a Purna Yoga, the Integral Path, as it includes all of man and consequently all of life in its comprehensive scope. To be sure, such a grand objective as this is beyond human means to reach. It is only the World-Power which has initiated the Movement that can lead it to its victorious culmination.

In the context of this aim of our Yoga, liberation of the individual soul, personal *mukti*, ceases to be the sole object. It is indeed indispensable, but only as a necessary and inevitable step. For without the central transcendence of the triple rule of the lower nature governed by Ignorance, no divine change is possible.

*   *   *

The first truth the sadhaka of this Yoga has to perceive is that all is the Divine, the One Brahman. He permeates all orders of existence. He is there in every creature, in every point of Space and in every moment of Time, supporting all as the *sad ātman*, an impersonal Self. All are Names and Forms on the bosom of this Self.

This realisation of an impersonal divine Existence deepens further into a second realisation in which one sees the Divine not only supporting and containing but also embodying itself in all things. Not only are all things in the Self, but the Self too is in all of them. It is That which makes the Names and Forms alive and real.

And there is a third, the crowning realisation to follow: above all there is the fact of an infinite Divine Personality, the Supreme Purusha, who transcends both the world of Names and Forms and the Impersonal Atman supporting them. It is He who has put out this universe from the infinitude of His being and who presides over it in the Lila of His manifestation.

The whole world-existence changes its hue. It is no more a battlefield of contraries; it is realised to be a variegated self-extension of the Divine Being in His waves of Light, Beauty and Bliss which strike under certain conditions as their very opposites. From Him radiate all these multiplications in Creation and it is in Him also that we find our oneness with others. He is the Lord in whose sovereign sway the sadhaka has to awaken and grow. It is to this Supreme Person that you have to deliver yourself for the completion of your life's mission.

If you would have the Master assume the reins of your being in his celestial hands you must surrender yourself to Him absolutely. Absolutely: neither in the mind, nor in the heart nor even in the body shall there be any reservation. All is to be given in a sacred offering. True, complete surrender is not possible in a day. Still one can begin with a whole-hearted *saṁkalpa*, an attitude, a will to surrender imposed on the entire being. No egoistic demand, however faint, no personal preference, however masked, shall be allowed to taint the purity of this consecration. All dualities must be renounced and all existence embraced as an expression of the One Divine. If you thus give yourself up wholly into His hands, the way is clear for the working of His Lila through you and in you.

When this is done there is no need of a formal discipline, *kriyā*. For it is the Divine who takes up and effectuates the Yoga. And besides, the utmost that man could do by his own effort is nothing compared to what is possible for His mighty Shakti.

Once the initial surrender to the Lord is made, the next step is to stand aside and observe the working of His Shakti. The complex movements of its process, now taking up a few ends here, now changing over to other threads there, unsettling the established round of nature,—all these and many more appear to land one in the very heart of chaos and bewilder the anticipating human mind. A quiet strong faith in the intelligence and the ultimate effectivity of the Higher Power at work is required of the sadhaka. Whatever is done within or without, it is the work of the Shakti offered to the Lord as a *yajña* of which the sadhaka is only the *yajamāna*. As the *yajamāna*, he holds the *ādhāra*, sees the sacrifice progress and tastes the fruit given to him. Not involved in the movement as a doer, he perceives the true nature and the extent of his *ādhāra*. He awakens too to the yet concealed regions of his being where the divine part of himself dwells—regions where abound masses of knowledge and the seas of *ānanda*—and he learns to let their revelation glide into an overt participation in his life-progression.

*   *   *

The sadhana of Purna Yoga has many lines of movement. But the most effective start is made by offering to the Divine the fruit of your actions. To give up the fruit of action means you do not perform actions for the particular fruits you expect of them; you do what comes to you ordained by the Master, *kartavyam karma*, regardless of the results. Whatever the results, they are given by God and you receive them with trust in His Wisdom.

Next, you surrender not only the fruit but the actions themselves to the Lord. You realise that you are not the doer. You perceive that it is really Prakriti, the executive Power of the Divine that is doing all action at the command of the Lord. It is He who determines the action through your *svabhāva* and it is the Prakriti who executes it. Once you realise this truth in the depths of your being,

16

neither action nor the results of action can bind you. Sri Aurobindo speaks of three stages in the growth of this knowledge :

first, when you surrender the initiative to the Master of your being and act as He directs;

second, when you believe that in the heart of all beings there is God moving them by his Maya of three Gunas and are able to perceive that you are really not the worker at all but it is the machinery of the three Gunas that does all works. By steady dissociation from the Gunas you stand above them in your central poise, the Purusha, and in time the Prakriti too will be free from their mechanical hold;

third, when the very Gunas, of which the Prakriti is constituted, undergo a transforming change. Sattva passes into Jyoti, pure illumination, Tamas into Shanti, infinite Calm and Rajas into Tapas, a divine Force. Whatever action proceeds from such a foundation of a new harmony will be, indeed, an undeflected expression of the will of the Purusha, one with the Will of God. A vast and mighty Force will be found moving and acting in you, possessing your mind, your heart, your very body, and you yourself will be one centre of the divine Dynamism.

It is indispensable for this liberation that you should be totally free from desire, *spṛhā,* which creates longing and attachment to things, from duality, *dvandva,* which forges on the being the clamps of attraction and repulsion, love and hate, from egoism, *ahaṇkāra*, which creates a false identification with things resulting in one's bondage to them. All these take their characteristic expression in the workings of the three Gunas of Tamas, Rajas and Sattva,—the most dangerous being the deceptive formulations of the Sattva Guna,—and are the enemies of self-surrender.

These processes are worked out by the Divine Shakti in its own rhythm with its own pace and stress varying with each individual need. All that is demanded of you is a continual remembrance, a constant assent to the workings of the Yoga Shakti with an unshakable faith and a vigilant perseverance. For the path is long, the Goal is high. It is nothing less than the acceleration of centuries of evolution into a few years of Yoga, the transformation of your entire human nature into a divine nature. Yet it is not your own puny will and effort but the infinite Shakti of the Almighty that is charged with the task and whatever the time taken, whatever the failings in the instrumental nature, its fulfilment is inevitable. The reliance here is on God and God does not fail even though man in his stumbling steps may.

These, then, are the four aids for the *siddhi* of this yoga :

S'āstra, the teaching of *sarvam khalu idam brahma*, All is Brahman, and *ātma samarpaṇa*, total self-surrender to the Lord of all;

Utsāha, zeal in pursuing the path with constant assent and remembrance;

Guru, the Teacher who is God Himself or the person who embodies Him to the disciple;

Kāla, Time, the duration of which is ultimately decided in the all-knowing Wisdom of the Master of all Yoga.

The Superman

FOR a sadhaka of the supramental Yoga, as indeed of all Yoga, it is indispensable to have beforehand a right understanding of the nature of the Goal of the path he is to tread. He should know, as precisely as possible, the full content of the Ideal, its implications immediate and eventual, so that no effort is misdirected or wasted, no turn taken that would defeat the very purpose of the Journey.

The aim of this Yoga is to exceed the boundaries of the imperfect mind in man and to enliven in him a principle which is free from the limitations of mind, a faculty which is above the mind,—the supermind. Man is to grow into a superman.

Now what exactly is meant by superman?

It goes without saying that a superman is not, as is commonly conceived or misconceived, simply a glorified edition of the ordinary man. A man whose powers and capacities are raised to an uncommon degree, towering high above his less fortunate fellow beings, dominating them by virtue of his superior might—this is the figure of the superman popularised by vitalist thinkers like Nietzsche.

Such a man, it will be noted, remains still a man. Only his faculties have an enlarged sway; they continue to be centred round his ego which is now much more exaggerated. He is a veritable titan, an Asura, whose role in the cosmic evolution is happily past. The superman of our conception is one who has cultivated and perfected in their fullest amplitude and height the essential powers of his being in all its ranges of body, life, mind and soul but at the same time has purged himself of all deformations of ego and ignorance and passed into godhead. He has risen above the reign of nature and enthroned himself in the freedom of the soul from where he governs her activities. He is the master of his own being, *svarāt*.

He too governs the lives of others but in another sense. He is one with them in the secrecies of their being, feels their heart-beats as his own and pours his energies for their advancement. Freed from the bonds of the separative ego, he expands in his consciousness gathering into its fold the wide universe around. He holds all in his clasp, not of power, but of love. He receives in his illumined being the movements of those around and returns them uplifted and charged with his transmuting vibrations which exert an incessant pressure on his environs moulding them in the likeness of the Truth of his living. He is the world-ruler, *samrāṭ*.

He is no more subject to the law of Division which is characteristic of the rule of mind. In him the several principles of Existence e.g., Knowledge, Love, Power, Unity, do not clash and seek to suppress each other in their drive for exclusive expression as they do in the mind-governed domain of man. They develop, each into its fullness, and find their completion in the fulfilment of all. All see each other as the common petals of a budding rose. The many notes struck by them fall into a rich harmony and he reproduces in himself the rhythms of the cosmic harp in the hands of God.

This and no other is the significance of the superman. To this end must man work with a singleness of purpose, exercising his will enlightened by the growing light of the soul at every step, to eliminate all that belongs to the lower order of life and to choose what leads to the higher, however difficult and arduous the course may be. But is he free to choose? Is man not, more truly, a leaf driven hither and thither by the gusts of universal forces? Is he not just a creature under the goad of Karma, Fate, forged by himself and by others?

*   *   *

There is, says Sri Aurobindo, a truth in Fate, in determinism. There is also, he adds, a truth in Free-will. Both are two movements of one Cosmic Energy put out by the Divine Shakti at work. The universe is an expression of a Will and all in it follows the lines of that Will for the execution of its Purpose. In this sense all is determined. But the Will works through a hundred currents of its own formulation as Power, Energy that is many-tiered. In the individual it works most effectively through his sense of freedom, freedom to choose and act. This freedom of the individual is a device of the All-Will to effectuate itself. The will of the individual is a segment of the Universal Will and what it works out is ultimately just what is assigned to it in the larger Plan of the One Will.

And yet, within certain limits the individual is free to choose. Even the compulsive factors in Nature, Heredity and Environment, which Modern Science emphasises to underline the rigid law of causation governing this material world, are only elements that are provided by an All-seeing Intelligence for the free choice of the soul at every graded step of its evolutionary career. Once chosen these factors come into their own operation, call it by whatever name you will. But it is the soul that chooses initially; it is again the soul that chooses its own destiny in the future by means of the Karma it puts out at every moment consciously.

The individual will is a part of the Universal Will and the secret of progress lies in the discovery of harmony between the two. As long as one chooses to act by one's own ego-will regardless of the demands of the greater Will there is friction, struggle and even catastrophe. But as one learns to identify oneself and make oneself Its instrument the friction dissolves and a harmonious working is ensured. To awaken to this role of the instrument is then the first necessity.

* * *

To the seeker of the truth of this Manifestation of the Divine, all work is work for the Divine and by the Divine. He perceives that for each work there is the Master of the Work, the Worker and the Instrument. He knows himself to be neither the Master nor the Worker. He is only the instrument. He equips himself as a ready and willing instrument whose sole aim is to serve as a perfect channel for the divine execution and whose whole joy lies in the privilege of being so chosen. He learns to feel the inmost law of his nature, sets all the members of his being in tune with this demand of the soul and grows into a joyous conscious instrument of the real Worker who is none other than Nature.

That Nature is All-Nature of which his own nature is a special movement. Hers is the one Force that works and effectuates simultaneously in the individual and in the universe. The sadhaka awakens to this fact of One Nature within and without and gradually identifies himself with the infinite Force of All-Nature. As his consciousness widens and deepens in this Knowledge, he becomes aware that it is not for herself that all work is done by Nature but for the One who is her Lord.

He discovers the poise of the Lord on the heights of his being even as he comes to recognise the dynamics of the Executrix-Nature in his own.

It is only when he knows and begins to live this triple truth of the Instrument, the Worker and the Master in his own being that man shall have the full joy of work, his share in the Lila of Manifestation.

The Letters

OF all the writings of Sri Aurobindo the most important from the standpoint of *sādhanā*, practice of yoga, are his Letters. His correspondence covers a large variety of subjects : Yoga, Philosophy, Literature, Art, Occultism, Astrology, Sociology, International affairs etc., etc. Aspirants for spiritual life, practitioners of his Yoga within the Ashram and outside, put their difficulties and doubts before him and sought his guidance and help. Experiences, visions, dreams were submitted for interpretation. Learned men and professional philosophers posed searching queries on fine points in the metaphysics of his gospel of the Life Divine. Disciples who found poetic inspiration welling up in them in the course of the Yoga sent their efforts for his scrutiny. At times even mundane matters and opinions of men in public life were placed before him for comment. And so it went on. He used to deal with most of the letters himself, meticulously, and for a considerable number of years it took a good many hours daily[1] to deal with all this volume

[1] *Vide* Sri Aurobindo's own remarks in this connection :
" The volume of correspondence is becoming enormous and it takes

of correspondence. At its peak there were more than a hundred letters every day. Many of his letters in reply were later compiled, either in full or in extracts, under suitable titles and issued in book-form from time to time.[1] Recently a comprehensive collection of his letters dealing with Yoga has been brought out in the Sri Aurobindo International Centre of Education Series.[2] And it is with the letters on Yoga that we are concerned in our present study.

Most of these letters were written to sadhaks of the Integral Yoga, in response to their queries and seekings for guidance. Developments and difficulties in the day-to-day course of the sadhana were placed before the Guru by the disciples and he wrote to them explaining, clarifying things, and

---

me all the night and a good part of the day—apart from the work done separately by the Mother who has also to work the greater part of the night in addition to her day's work."

"I have to spend twelve hours over the ordinary correspondence, numerous reports etc. I work three hours in the afternoon and the whole night up to six in the morning over this." (*Sri Aurobindo on Himself and on the Mother*).

[1] *The Riddle of this World, Lights on Yoga, Bases of Yoga, More Lights on Yoga, Elements of Yoga, Letters (First, Second, Third and Fourth Series), Life-Literature-Yoga, Correspondence with Sri Aurobindo* (by Nirodbaran), I & II series.

[2] *On Yoga*, Vol. II, Tomes 1 & 2.
This is, naturally, not yet exhaustive ; letters are still being collected and edited. They are being published, as they get ready, in some of the periodicals of the Ashram, viz., *The Advent, Mother India*, Annual Numbers of *Sri Aurobindo Circle*, Bombay.

what is more, he used such occasions to communicate his special help, through the medium of the written word and otherwise, in order to meet the situation and speed up the progress. And these communications were a source of inspiration and helpful pointers on the Path to others as well. As he himself says:

"If I have given importance to the correspondence, it is because it was an effective instrument towards my central purpose—there are a large number of sadhaks whom it has helped to awaken from lethargy and begin to tread the way of spiritual experience, others whom it has carried from a small round of experience to a flood of realisations, some who have been absolutely hopeless for years who have undergone a conversion and entered from darkness into an opening of light . . . for the majority of those who wrote there has been real progress. No doubt also it was not the correspondence in itself but the Force that was increasing in its pressure on the physical nature which was able to do all this, but a canalisation was needed, and this served the purpose.[1]

It is not necessary to add that the letters were not answers in the usual intellectual way but 'answers from higher spiritual experience, from a deeper source of knowledge and not lucubrations of the logical intellect trying to co-ordinate its

---

[1] *Sri Aurobindo on Himself and on the Mother.*

ignorance'.[1] In them we see Sri Aurobindo not in the role of the Prophet of the high Philosophy of the Life Divine, nor even as the High Priest ushering in a New Age by means of a Poorna Yoga holding in itself all the essentials of the past spiritual effort of humanity and forging a new Dynamism, but as the Master with a supreme understanding of human nature and its countless foibles, with an endless compassion for its cry for help, ever ready to support, guide, and lead the seeker with an infinite patience along the steep path of Yoga. Nothing is too small, nothing too profane to claim his attention. His Yoga touches life at every point and no part of it is outside his scope. As a result, we have in these Letters a most comprehensive body of practical knowledge not only invaluable for those living an inner life of the spirit but an equally reliable guide for a better, harmonious and enlightened conduct of the general life.

*   *   *

Though it is true that each individual has his own line of spiritual growth and what is valid for one need not be so for another, yet there are certain fundamental truths which are common to all types of sadhana. And this is particularly true in the

---

[1] *Sri Aurobindo on Himself and on the Mother.*

case of sadhaks of the same Yoga. Whatever the individual variations in the experience of the Yoga-process, the broad governing Truth is the same. It is with this background that we have to approach the Letters of Sri Aurobindo for a helpful study of his Yoga.

The Object
of Integral Yoga

TO begin with, what is the object of the Integral Yoga developed by Sri Aurobindo?

The object is, first, to grow from the normal limited human consciousness into a higher, wider Divine Consciousness.

Next, this Divine Consciousness with all that it contains,—Peace, Light, Joy, Knowledge,—is to be progressively brought into a direct functioning in our external nature in order to totally change that nature into its own higher illumined term, the Supernature.

The purpose of this transformation is to manifest the Divine in our life. And of this manifestation our personal liberation is a part—only a part, though an indispensable one. This manifestation of the Divine in our life implies a realisation and a sequent radiation of the Divine Consciousness not in the soul alone but equally in all the different parts of the being. What is aimed at is a complete union with the Divine on all the planes of one's being. The mind, the life, the body, the soul, all must be equally filled with the Divine Presence and be effective centres for the outpouring of the Divine Power in the universe.

Or, to put it differently, the Integral Yoga has three clear objects in view:

First, the realisation of the Divine within one-self—the individual realisation.

Next, a felt seeing of the One Divine all around in the universe, the Divine which is identical with one's own Self—the cosmic realisation.

And third, an ascension into an order of the Reality which stands above both the individual and the universal manifestation, but bases them both —the transcendental realisation.

Each of these realisations must be attained and integrated within one's being so as to be simultaneously active and the miracle of the triple manifestation of God[1] is repeated in every individual frame: each man grows into his godhead.

It may be asked what the special feature and necessity of this Yoga is. After all God is One and there are a thousand paths to reach Him. What does it matter which path you take? What is important is that you reach Him whatever be the path.

DISTINCTION FROM OTHER PATHS

Generally speaking, the goal of all the paths of Yoga is *mukti*, liberation. The world is a transient phenomenon, or an illusion; if it is not totally

---

[1] Individual, Universal and Transcendent.

an illusion, it is definitely an inferior order of existence.[1] Limitation, incapacity and death are its
badge. The one aim of the awakened man must
be to get out of this round of pain and pleasure,
life and death and effect a release into a blissful
or an ineffable Beyond, call it Brahman, call it
Nirvana. But in Sri Aurobindo's Teaching the
Universe is as real as the Divine of which it is a
willed Emanation. It is not a falsity imposed upon
the Truth of Brahman. Nor is it something inferior.
It is a self-formulation, *as yet imperfect*, of the
manifesting Godhead. And the sole object of the
Yoga of Sri Aurobindo is to complete this out-
flowering of the Divine Consciousness on earth. It
aims at a fulfilment of the Divine Intention, first
in the life of the individual and then in the life of the
collectivity. It gives a meaning to the life on earth
which is not a whit less significant—perhaps it is
more—than life in the heavens in the scheme of
Creation.

Aiming as they do to reject life in this appa-
rently transitory and unhappy world, the other
yogas generally seek to realise the Self, the Atman,
behind or above the mind-led life of the body, and
through it disappear into the Vast Impersonality of
the Great Self or into Nirvana, extinction. That is
to say, the way is one of withdrawal from the line

[1] Or, in conceptions like the Christian, life on earth is only a
preparatory stage to an eternal existence elsewhere—heaven or
hell—after death.

of manifestation of which this earth forms a crucial part. The Integral Yoga on the other hand, keeps to the evolutionary line of ascent in the Manifestation. The self within is to be realised ; but that is only the first step. After attaining to union with this self, one has to effect an enlargement of the consciousness to arrive at an identity with the larger Self, the Universal Atman and embrace the totality of Existence supported by It. This is further followed by an ascension into the dynamics of the Divine Knowledge, Power, Bliss—an aspect which reveals itself to the seeker beyond the summits of the spiritualised mind, on the planes of the Supermind. And it is these verities of the Divine Existence that justify the human aspiration for perfection of life on earth. It is they that shall bring into overt expression the full Nature of the Divine, hitherto at the back of the manifestation, and confirm and complete the movement for the revelation of the Divine Truth in human life.

The aim is different ; the direction is different ; the process too is different in important details. For instance, in the other yogas one is not called upon to subject one's nature to a transmuting change. It is enough if the nature is silenced or modified enough to prevent its being a drag or a block to the inner progress of the soul godward. Even after the realisation is achieved, no special attention is paid to the outer nature. It goes on in its mechanical round carried on the impetus of past

Karma and drops away at the death of the body leaving the soul completely free. But it is not so in this yoga. Each part of the nature, submissive or recalcitrant, has to change; it has to leave its moorings in ignorance and allow itself to be recast into its higher potential. The whole of the external nature, including the physical body, must be made supple and pure enough to hold and respond spontaneously to the Divine Consciousness housed in it.

Again, in this yoga, there is no suppression or stoppage of the flow of life energies or the legitimate activity of the senses. They continue to function in full but in an enlightened spirit imbued with the growing Light, Power and Delight of the Divine Truth. Not asceticism but a radiant plenitude of life is the Way. In the ways of the Vedanta, it is enough for the inner Purusha to attain union with the Divine; in those of the Tantra, what is required is an effective identification with the Shakti, indidual and cosmic, and that gives the release. But here both are combined. The Realisation in the consciousness of the Purusha has to spread to the Prakriti. The Purusha regains his mastery over Prakriti and both together lift their human embodiment to an altogether new altitude in the scale of human Evolution.

Basic Requisites of Integral Yoga

TO take up this yoga, one must first feel the need for it. There should be a *Call* for the higher life. And the call must be genuine, must proceed from the depths of the being. Impulsions from the surfaces of the mental or of the vital personality, either as a result of some dissatisfaction in life or ambition—under whatever camouflage—could never be a sufficient reason. They do not last for long and there comes the inevitable flag, after the initial push is spent out. One must feel a real need to change the ordinary way of living into a higher. There should be a thirst for the Divine as the fish, in the apt imagery, thirsts for water. The demand must be of the soul with a sustained pressure on the mind and the vital to seek and share the change. Again the novice must make sure of the type of spiritual life for which he has affinity. For this Integral Yoga there must be an aspiration in the whole of one's being, not only in the mind and the soul, but in the life-being and the body too, to be reborn in the dynamic truth of the Spirit and to participate in the Divine's manifestation. If the call is only for Mukti, liberation, then there is no need to choose this difficult path of transformation. There are other traditional paths for that purpose.

Next is *Sincerity*. And by sincerity is meant a constant readiness and effort to lift up all the parts and all the movements of one's being, in consonance with the truth of one's seeking. It is not enough if the sincerity is there at the centre, in the mind or in the heart. It should spread to all the parts of one's being so that each acts spontaneously on the same basis and for the same aim. The whole being must be true to the Ideal it has set out to realise. Nothing foreign to that should be allowed to touch, much less express itself in any of its thinkings or doings.

There must be *Faith*, faith in the reality of the Divine, faith in the Path that leads to the Divine, and faith in the Grace that carries one to the Goal. Here too it is not enough if there is only a belief or a certain adherence in the thought i.e. the mind. There is required an entire faith, a dynamic conviction in all the parts of one's being. Sri Aurobindo speaks of four kinds of faith : the mental faith which dispels all doubts and prepares for true knowledge ; the vital faith which automatically repels onslaughts of the adverse forces and builds up an effective instrumentation of the divine Will and action ; the physical faith which sustains the body amidst all its tribulations of suffering, illness and inertia and silently prepares for the reception of the higher consciousness in the material base; and lastly the psychic faith which draws a direct touch of the Divine Influence and leads to a joyous surrender to and intimacy with the Divine.

And of course there must be an *Aspiration.* The aspiration for the Divine has to be active, growing, setting aflame each centre of the being so that in due course the whole system is one tongue of Agni reaching out to the Heavens Supreme. This aspiration, to be effective, must needs be accompanied by a corresponding will to translate it into action. This conjoint movement manifests itself in the mind as a thirst for and growth into Knowledge, in the vital being as an urge shaping into a dynamic activity dedicated to the Divine, in the heart as a welling up of the emotions of love and devotion, all in adoration of the Divine. Even the body calls for and yields to a settling calm and peace in its very texture so as to form a firm pedestal for the rising structure.

All this is rendered possible by another means, *Surrender.* Surrender is a willed delivering of one-self to another, here the Divine. In this Yoga, starting from a part which most easily tends to so surrender itself, the movement gradually spreads over to the other parts making them all fall in line, so that the whole of oneself is placed in the hands of the Divine in absolute trust and confidence. This surrender is of two kinds, passive and active. It is active when the individual will is sought to be harmonised and identified with the divine Will at every step—this is what is called consecration—and there is a conscious effort to accept only what is divine and reject what is undivine. It is passive when no will is exercised, but the entire being is kept in a state of readiness to be acted upon by the Divine Will. This latter way is more difficult and unless one is very vigilant one gets bogged in tamasic inertia or becomes a plaything of the forces of the lower nature.

That brings us to the next requisite, *Vigilance,* vigilance to spot out the opposite and wrong currents as they try to enter, to feel the right and upward movements as they set in and to tend them in the proper direction. This is indispensable so long as the sadhana has not been completely taken charge of by the Higher Power and personal effort has its part to play. Once the direction is taken up by the higher Agency, there is an automatic action of the psychic being within replacing the labour of mental vigilance.

For success in any spiritual life, especially in a Yoga as this where one aims to participate in the dynamic manifestation of the Divine, it is essential that the *ego* must be dissolved. Ego is a false front of the real individuality within and unless that is removed the true self cannot come into its own. Human ego has many disguises, many centres of operation and aggrandisement. There is the tamasic ego of wallowing in inertia, weakness and ignorance in a spirit of loud helplessness, a vital or rajasic ego of the sense of one's power and dominion, a sattvic ego of one's superior wisdom and moral righteousness, even a spiritual ego of sainthood. Each and every one of these forms of ego must be exposed and broken. This is a preliminary and yet a fundamental step to be taken before one can be secure on the path. A full recognition of one's limitations, awareness of one's imperfections, and a becoming humility before the Vastness of the Divine that seeks to manifest, are of great help in the elimination of the ego which is truly a formidable enemy of the soul.

These are the main requisites for sadhana on the part of the individual. His personal effort must base itself and proceed on these lines, for personal effort there has to be in the beginning and for a long time, till the initiative passes from him into the hands of the Guiding Power ; even then, a continued state of receptivity and constant assent to its workings by the sadhaka is demanded. All these, however, constitute only one side of the endeavour. For, whatever may be the position in disciplines like the Advaitic or the Buddhist, in this Yoga the main burden rests with the Divine Power to whom an entire surrender is made. It is the Shakti that has first to assent to the sacrifice, the Divine Grace that has to accept and second the effort of the aspirant. That Grace is to be invoked and waited upon. For ultimately it is not the personal exertions of the human will but the uplifting move and the transforming touch of the Divine Grace that carries one over every obstacle and steadily changes the lower nature into the higher. And the Divine Grace is here manifest in the benign Person of the Guru, our Lord Sri Aurobindo and the Blissful Divine Mother who are pouring out in their compassion streams of Grace in abundance like the sempiternal Indra of the Veda raining the plenteous Waters of Heaven.

There have been disputes among scholars whether it is *tapasyā*, personal effort, that achieves or it is really the Grace that effects the result. In Sri Aurobindo's Yoga there is no room for any such doubt. Both are necessary; they are two sides of the working Truth. Divine Grace, surely, but for the Grace to be fully manifest the recipient should be ready. His being has got to be prepared, made pure, supple and sufficiently strong to receive, contain and collaborate with its workings. Otherwise the Breath of Grace will just pass by awaiting its Hour in the future. As the Mother says: "For transformation, Grace and aspiration are equally important. Grace comes first but if aspiration does not answer to It no progress is possible."

Foundations of Sadhana

ONE can begin the sadhana in any part of the being that is more awake than the others and seeks a higher direction. In some it is the heart that is astir and longs for the Divine Beloved; for them the most natural way is the Way of Love and Devotion. In some it is the mind that is ardent and searches for a Truth that is more satisfying than any it has known thitherto; for them is the Way of Meditation and Knowledge. In others it is the will, the life-dynamism that is dissatisfied with the normal round of activity and seeks to yoke itself to a higher Purpose and serve the Lord of All; for them is the Way of Works.

But whichever the Way one takes to in order to transcend the ordinary nature of humanity and grow into the heights and expanses of supernature, it is essential that the foundations of the sadhana are laid firm. Unless one prepares the base of the *ādhāra* strong enough to bear the incessant pressure of the Yoga Force at work for change, for growth, for reconstitution of the very texture of the being as in our Yoga, there is every danger of failure or breakdown on the way. The ordinary mind and the vital nature of man are apt to lose their balance and go off at a tangent once they are released—in the course of yoga—from the limitations to which they are normally subject; they may get over-whelmed by the descents of joy, power and light that greet the yogin on the path. The physical body itself, unless it is freed of its obscurity and rendered supple, may not respond pliantly to the demands of the Yoga-Shakti. To avert these dangers it is indispensable that the sadhaka first lays a strong foundation for the structure to come.

The very first step in laying the proper foundation, says Sri Aurobindo, is to acquire a Quiet in the being. Quiet means a state of mind in which there is no restlessness, no movement of anxiety or similar emotion which keeps a constant tenseness in the being and to that extent interferes with the opening of the being to the Higher Consciousness and obstructs the smooth and conscious reception of the incoming vibrations of the Higher Force or the outflowings of the soul within.

This quietude of the mind, *acañcalatā*, is to be acquired, built up with vigilance and will. It can be said to be established when there is no habitual restlessness, no incessant movement keeping the mind in a whirl. Though a negative condition, it is the first step leading to the next, the Calm, *sthiratā*. Calm is a more positive state in which there is a kind of tranquillity which is not disturbed by movement on the surface. Disturbances may come and pass but they move on the surface; the mind is serene. Sri Aurobindo describes two kinds of Calm : the negative calm where there is no contrary movement; the positive calm which solidly resists all movements that seek to disturb.

A still more positive condition is when there is entry of Peace, *s̓ānti*, in the being. It carries with it a sense of solidity, harmony and deliverance with a quiet Ananda permeating its vibrations. In such a state there can be no real disturbance which can affect the secure poise of the being.

The being is to be gradually taught to grow into these conditions of Quiet, Calm and Peace. Unless it frees itself from its habitual turmoil and naturalises these into its system, there can be no secure holding of the riches of the Spirit which one calls down into oneself by aspiration and will and which the Grace sanctions.

The most effective way to begin is mentally to conceive a Silence which is at the back of all movement. After all, thoughts are not the texture of the mind. Thoughts pass, other thoughts come and they too flit across some silent and immobile background of the mind. A repeated suspension of the thought-movement, and an increasing awareness of the Silence behind, effects the needed opening and the Silence begins to take hold of the mind. It is in this condition that Calm and Peace settle themselves. Here too, there are two kinds of silence. One, in which there is absolutely no movement in the inner consciousness; there is no reaction at all to activity in the external being; this is the passive silence. The other is the active silence in which from out of the Silence there goes out a powerful force of action without leaving a ripple within.

For true Peace to settle in the being there must be this stillness, the silence which prepares a state of utmost receptivity; it keeps the vessel empty. But this peace is not static. It is active and spreads to the other parts of the being as they begin to accept it, though initially it may enter through the mind. It has a purifying action wherever it goes and thus builds up a developing condition of purity which is an indispensable factor for progress in sadhana.

Purity is an equally essential part of the foundation. Naturally, by purity is not meant physical cleanliness. Nor is it only a moral rectitude of the kind spoken of in the Dharma Sastras. Purity, in Sri Aurobindo's sense, means an exclusive opening to the Divine alone; it implies the total rejection of all influences alien to the Divine. A sole fidelity to the Divine is what purity means in our sadhana. And Peace helps in the growth of this purity inasmuch as disturbing and foreign movements are automatically rejected from a state of Peace. Peace admits only those movements which are akin to its nature, nourish it and thrive in it. Further, inner Peace lessens the necessity of outer contacts and minimises the intrusion of external influences.

Next comes Equality, *samatā.* The normal human mind and vital nature are always apt to identify themselves with men and events, forces and circumstances, as they impinge upon the person, and get lost in the rush of their emotions and passions. For a sadhaka it is necessary that he should detach himself from the current of happenings; he has to learn gradually to stand back from the rush of Prakriti and observe things aloof from them. That way he acquires a dispassion, a growing equanimity which faces men and events in the world without getting helplessly involved in them. All contacts are received in an equable and unmoved status by the being and the utmost is made of each circumstance for an ordered and rapid growth of the evolving consciousness.

It is of course difficult to attain to this state of calm equality within a short time. A fund of patience and a steady will, persistent in the face of all opposition and difficulty, to acquire and make this inner equanimity a natural poise of the being is demanded of the sadhaka.

And lastly there must be a spiritual atmosphere in which the sadhana can thrive. If one can get it, for instance, in the environs of the Guru, nothing could be better. If not, one must create the spiritual air around oneself and live in it. And that is possible because the atmosphere one carries is always a reflection of the state of one's inner consciousness.

The Way of Works

ONE cannot but work, declares the Lord in the Gita. At every moment of our life we work in some way or other; we put out some energy consciously or unconsciously in the field of Karma. And where there is work there is usually a motive, a propelling factor that operates ceaselessly till the object is achieved and another replaces it. Normally the motive for work is based upon one's ego, self-interest, self-preservation, self-aggrandisement, and even when it extends beyond the range of one's personal self, it is still for interests related to the larger extensions of that self in the family, the society, the nation etc., or it is for the expression and affirmation of one's own ideas and ideals. Work so motivated and dictated by the demands of the ego continually forges fresh chains of Karma that keep the soul perpetually bound. For this reason, most spiritual disciplines counsel a gradual dissociation of the Purusha from the round of works, leaving the irreducible minimum to be performed by the mechanical Nature, Prakriti. In our Yoga, however, works are recognised as a God-given means of evolution and self-expression and valued as such. It is the motive that is sought to be changed. The usual impulsion based on the ego of the individual is to be replaced by a motive that derives from a deeper or higher origin, the psychic or the spiritual being. In this Path, works are directed to the Divine, performed for the Divine and even originated by the Divine. The individual remains but an instrument, a channel. Work is first used as a means for the establishment and the growth of self-dedication and consecration to the Divine and then utilised as a field for the expression of the Divine Consciousness that is being gradually realised and imbibed by the sadhaka in the course of his sadhana in works.

In order to convert work into a means of sadhana one begins by offering to the Divine the work that falls to one's share. Once it is dedicated to the Divine, work acquires a sacred character. It cannot be done in a light manner ; sincerity demands an appropriate order of application. An offering to the Divine has to be necessarily as perfect as possible and commensurate with his devotion ; there is an earnest attempt on the part of the sadhaka to do the work in a spirit of loving consecration. Every little part of it gains importance, no detail can now be left out imperfectly done. Further, it is no more the kind of work that truly matters but the spirit in which it is done. As the spirit of consecration grows, there is a happiness in the being, a stream of delight from the emotional and the psychic being converting the whole working into a rite of joyous progression in the Pathway to the Divine.

And in this process of doing one's best to make of work a worthy offering to the Adored, there is an automatic concentration of faculties and convergence of energies towards the One to whom the entire work is consecrated. Of course all this is not done in a day. It is not at once easy to remember continually the Divine to whom the offering is made. One forgets again and again and the mechanical habit of working asserts itself. Sri Aurobindo states encouragingly that to start with, it is enough to remember before the work is begun and to remember again with gratitude after the work is done. In between there are moments when one remembers; these should be steadily increased; if necessary, one can inwardly withdraw for a moment now and then, remember and renew the offering. If the initial will for consecration is sincere, one finds in the course of time that there are, as it were, two parts of oneself: one part engaged in work and the other silent, remembering the Divine. This calm and quiet being comes forward at moments when there is a suspension of the external preoccupation; but it should be possible for the sadhaka to be more and more aware of its supporting presence even during activity. Gradually, increasingly, one comes to experience that the whole of oneself is this quiet and gathered being with only its frontal part doing the work.

This is the beginning. The work is offered to the Divine, but not the results; they are sought after still on the basis of desire. The next step is to offer the fruits too to the Divine. Let the results be what the Divine determines, let me work irrespective of what they might be, leaving it to Him to make of them what He will. That is the attitude to be adopted by the sadhaka. If sincerely accepted and cultivated, this attitude gradually eliminates the claim and the domination of ego and desire and promotes a certain equality in the mind. For once both the work and its fruits are offered to the Divine, there is no straining for a particular personal result, no agitation of anxiety or fear of reverse; whatever the results they are taken as indicating the Divine Will. The human will becomes only the servant of the Divine Will.

To be the servant of the Divine is only the first step. To be an instrument is the next. For this purpose the sadhaka has to invoke the Divine Shakti to take up the work and do it through him. And for this to be possible there are a few minimum conditions to be fulfilled. In the first place, there must be a sufficient degree of purity in the being, especially in the vital and the mental energies; the claims and preferences of the ignorant mind and the habits of the ego-ridden life-being should not be allowed to interfere with the guidance and the working of the Higher Force. There has to be a steady and effective elimination of these impurities from the system. A sufficient measure of Equality and Quiet in the mind, in the face of all likes and dislikes, all contradictions and oppositions that assail the worker, is indispensable and that can be developed only on the basis of a strong Faith, faith that all is determined by the Sole Divine and in spite of appearances all leads in sum to the result intended by the Divine. Only in such a state of quiet faith can one become aware of the presence and working of a Higher Shakti, the Divine Consciousness and Force. And becoming aware, one has to open oneself—in the static as well as in the active condition—to that Consciousness and to no other influence. Then the Force to which one opens oneself begins to act, first in moments when one is receptive, then in stretches of receptive periods and then longer and longer. There is not only a constant guidance and impulsion to do what is to be done, but also a vigilant and forceful pulling back from what should not be done. The human will and energy are taken up by the Shakti which makes them its channel and through them executes its purpose. All the while, it will be noted, the human consciousness goes on receiving the impacts and the pressure of the Divine Consciousness and Force; on the human side from below there is a rigorous discipline processing the system in the way of concentration, purification, dedication and receptivity to the Divine. All work becomes a sadhana to grow into the rising altitudes of the Divine Consciousness and receive the incoming Force and Illumination in one's own person.

Work is not only a means of ascent to the highest but more. Work is simultaneously a means to express what one acquires by way of enlightenment of will and power, increasing purity of motive and illumination of energy. In short, work becomes a field to bring out the inner gains and confirm them in the outer nature also by accustoming its faculties to express them infallibly. Further, once the individual is equipped as an instrument, the Divine Force that acts need not be limited in its dynamics by the imperfections of its nature. It can act in its own full power using the instrument as a readied medium. It may also—and usually does—train and perfect the instrument by acclimatizing it to the workings of its higher nature and naturalising in it the vibrations and movements of a higher Knowledge and Power. The sadhaka develops into a potent centre for the greater radiation of spiritual energy in the world.

The Way of Meditation

IT is possible to train the being to tune itself to the workings of the Divine Consciousness by another means, *dhyāna.*

Dhyana, commonly translated as Meditation, is of several kinds only one of which can be truly called Meditation. Sri Aurobindo analyses these different forms of Dhyana into four main kinds. There is first, meditation (*manana*) which is a dwelling of the mind on a line of thought or series of ideas constituting a single subject. The mind is allowed to flow into a channel of thought-activity centred around the object of meditation, which may be a Knowledge-Idea — say, the Divine as omnipresent, the Divine as one's own highest Self, the Divine as an Impersonal Power, the Divine as a Personal Deity with several attributes — or simply a Call to the Divine. The second is contemplation, a more concentrated direction of the mental faculties on a *single* Idea or Image or object. As a result of this concentration there arises in the mind, naturally, a knowledge of the object contemplated upon. There is a third kind, the Dhyana of self-observation, in which one stands back from the running activity of thoughts and only observes the nature of one's mind as shown by the thoughts. The fourth is the process by which the thoughts are steadily rejected and the mind kept more and more free from the turbidity of thoughts so as to provide a more or less empty vessel in which the Higher Consciousness may settle itself ; this is the Dhyana of liberation, liberation of the mind from its mechanical and inferior movements into purer altitudes giving it the freedom to think or not to think, the power to choose its thoughts or go beyond them.

Each of these forms of Dhyana has its own value in spiritual life. The individual chooses that which is most natural to him. It is also found in the course of sadhana that the same line of Dhyana may not be suitable at all times. Different Dhyana-processes may be called for at different stages of development and one should be supple enough to use whichever method is the most helpful during the period.

The central principle of Dhyana, it will be observed, is to summon the various faculties of the being, particularly the mental forces, which are usually spread out in innumerable directions, and gather them round the object of one's quest. Indeed, in an ideal condition the entire being stands naturally so gathered and mobilised around the Truth of its seeking all the time. But a long prior discipline is necessary to train the being in this direction and to accustom it to function in that poise for longer and longer periods before it settles in that position normally. And this discipline is what is called Dhyana, Meditation.

There are certain conditions which are very helpful in the beginning, external and internal. There should be, in the first place, a reasonable measure of solitude, a seclusion where one could be by oneself and meditate without fear of physical intrusion or interruption by others. The next condition is that the body must be trained to take up a position that is most helpful for the purpose of meditation. That position is ideal in which the body settles into a state of gathered immobility freeing the rest of the being from the pull of the physical frame and providing for it a firm and stable base. The sitting position is the best for in that one can continue the course of meditation for longer stretches of time undistracted by restlessness or tiredness in the body. The sitting position in which the spine is kept erect and the chest, the neck and the head held up straight is the best posture as it promotes stability and a healthy coursing of vitality in the body infusing fresh currents of life-energy in the mental and *prāṇic* organisms which are the leading participants in the meditation.

The very first difficulty one meets with the moment one begins to meditate is the rush of thoughts. Thoughts crowd in such a bewildering profusion that it looks as if there are more thoughts during meditation than at other times. But this is not quite so. The fact is, normally, men are so preoccupied with many other things that they are not conscious of the innumerable thoughts floating on the surface of the mind. When one prepares for meditation the mind is focussed in a narrower circle and the flow of thoughts comes to the notice more prominently than ever. Now there are ways of countering this invasion of thoughts.

One can stand back from the waves of thought and observe them without sanctioning or participating in them. There is no effort to reject or fight them. One simply stands back as a witness. Gradually for want of support from the active mind the thoughts begin to dwindle and peter away. Another way is to treat the thoughts as coming from outside and vigilantly check them when they try to enter the mind. Each thought is to be so detected and thrown out before it comes in or as soon as it is discovered. A third way is to treat the thoughts as foreign, as coming from Prakriti and for oneself to stand in the poise of the witness Purusha, without sanction, without approval or disapproval, aloof. This leads in time to a kind of bifurcation, a division in the mind — one part is quiet and watches, the other is the scene of crossing thoughts. It is possible afterwards to impose the quietude of the witness part on the part involved in the thought-movement. Yet another way is to ignore the movements of thoughts on the surface of the mind and to go within with a will, pursuing the object of meditation. This succeeds to the measure of the interest aroused in the mind : where it has interest there the mind turns. The best method, however, is to remember and invoke the Silence and Peace that stands at the back of all thought and movement. Whether at the back of our mind or behind the universal movements there is a supporting Silence, a Calm, a Peace. And the sadhaka should learn to mentally envisage it, invoke it and gently lay himself open to its entry. In course of time, this Calm and Silence makes itself felt and once it enters the mind, in whatever layer, the end of the rule of thoughts begins. It is this Silence and Peace that is to be regarded, concentrated upon, ignoring the activity of the surface mind. Sri Aurobindo points out that it is easier and more natural to let this Silence take hold of us than for us to enter into it. And as the Silence, the Peace, settles in the being, the consciousness gets readied to receive and assimilate what comes from above or within and opens to the reign of the Divine. The turbid contents of the human vessel—passions, desires and their reactions—are steadily replaced by a quiet joy, enlightened emotions and increasing purity.

The success of the meditation depends largely upon the sincerity and strength of the aspiration behind it. It is not duration but the intensity of the aspiring consciousness that is important. The Mother once observed that three minutes of intense aspiration is worth much more than hours of stagnant meditation. Fatigue is to be avoided at all costs : for with it concentration loses its power and the mind jades. Sri Aurobindo advises relaxation into meditation instead of concentration in such cases.

That brings us to other difficulties usually encountered in meditation. Frequently one is overcome by sleep. However, this sleep, it must be remembered, is not the usual kind of sleep. As a result of the pressure to go within, the consciousness as it withdraws from the external world tends to lapse by habit into sleep. But it is only a part of it that so sinks into sleep ; if there be sufficient fire of aspiration, the larger part of the consciousness is seen to be luminously active within, below or behind the layer of sleep. If the sleep were of the ordinary tamasic variety, it would not be possible for the body to hold itself for long in the erect posture of meditation.

Then there are the obstructions of forgetfulness, inertia and absorption into the mechanically repetitive habits of the mind ; they are best negatived by constant vigilance, ardour and a strong will in the effort. There are also the obstacles of restlessness, impatience, over-eagerness and violence of effort which soon tire and bring in depression. These are to be eliminated and replaced by patience, persistence and a quiet aspiration.

During meditation the consciousness (not merely the outer mind which is only a segment of it) is withdrawn from its usual activity of ceaseless reception of and response to external contacts and turned to its own larger expanse, whether inwards or upwards, which is more open to and in a way in contact with the Divine Consciousness. So turned and tuned, the limited human consciousness is exposed to the touches and workings of the Force of the Higher Consciousness which prepare and precipitate its change from the lower into the higher, from the human into the divine nature. This concentration of consciousness is usually done either in the head or in the heart. When the natural inclination is to seek the Divine within oneself, the concentration is done in the heart centre (in the middle of the chest, the cardiac centre) with a strong aspiration for an opening inward and realisation of the Divinity seated deep within. When the urge is to rise in one's consciousness above the bounds of the mind or to invoke the descent of the Peace above the mind, the concentration is done in the head. Such a concentration is indeed strenuous but the strain begins to disappear as one learns to 'lift the concentration above the brain-mind'.

Thus meditation puts the being of the sadhaka in a condition of increasing and conscious receptivity to the workings of the Yoga Shakti. As it deepens there is even a total forgetfulness of the external environment and outer nature. There is a steady settling in of peace, joy, light, knowledge and other inalienable powers of the Higher Consciousness in the inner mind and being of the practicant. In most lines of Yoga this condition, experienced uninterruptedly in the hours of Samadhi —the crown of Dhyana—, is stabilised and organised into a state of liberation in the inner being to the exclusion of the rest of oneself—the external nature in its triple formulation on the mental, vital and physical levels—under the rule of Ignorance. But in the Integral Yoga of Sri Aurobindo, care is taken to relate the inner realisation at every step to the outer nature. The ordinary consciousness which is sought to be completely stilled and immobilised into the state of Samadhi in the older Yogas, the Patanjala Yoga, for instance, is here quieted and into that quietude are brought down the powers of the Higher or Deeper Consciousness to change its very nature. The condition of receptivity and illumination realised during meditation is consciously prolonged even during other hours and made the base of all movements of active life. As one progresses inly, further effort is made to communicate and dynamise in terms of life the golden gains of Meditation.

The Way of Love

Love is the easiest key to open the Gates to the Divine. This is a love that wells up spontaneously from the depths of the heart, oozes out from every pore of the body at the very thought of the Divine Beloved. It is a love which is very different from what we call by the same name in human relationships. What passes for love in the ordinary world is really no love at all but a mixture of desire and self-interest masquerading under as attachment, affection, love. Its root is ego and the moment the return it expects fails to come there is a revolt; love is on its way to turn into hate. The love that we speak of in Yoga is totally different. And there too, usually, it is not there in the beginning but comes as a culmination of the movement of devotion, Bhakti.

Even Bhakti, says the Scripture, is not always an unmixed offering of the emotions to the Divine. There is a Bhakti of appeal for succour from distress, *ārta*; there is a Bhakti propelled by desire seeking its fulfilment from the Divine, *arthārthī*; there is a Bhakti which is the outcome of the thirst for knowledge of the Divine who attracts but is still

5

Unknown, the Bhakti of the *jijñāsu*. There is also a Bhakti which is the result of the Knowledge, *jñānam*, that the Divine is the Sole Lord of All. Whatever the nature of the initial Bhakti, it should be taken as a starting point and an effort made to gradually cleanse its content, purge it of its grosser motives and turn it more and more into purer channels leading towards selfless love. In this the seeker is helped by the very nature of Bhakti which whatever its original motive, apparent or real, comes into its own as it grows in his being and raises him repeatedly to the high peaks of utter gratitude, pure love and clean aspiration, all of which are doors of entry into the realm of Love.

The first movement of Bhakti is one of *adoration*. Usually this takes the form of some kind of external worship of the adored. The devotee tends to express his feeling of submission and reverence through physical means which is natural to a mind that normally dwells in the world of the physical senses. This worship has indeed its preparatory value. But to be truly effective in opening a way of contact and communication with the Divine who is worshipped, this outer mode of attendance must correspond to an inner feeling, a glad movement of surrender, a dependence felt within. The outer should be a means of expression, a support for the growth of an *inner adoration*. The inner gives life to the outer.

With the birth of this inner adoration Yoga

may be said to begin in right earnest. An inner life begins to take shape. The sense of submission and waiting upon the Divine with devotion—implied in the act of adoration—has certain practical consequences. There is an automatic action to keep the temple of one's being clean for the Divine. Thoughts and feelings turn into movements of seeking and prayer. The external life too comes to be moulded in tune with this inner ordering.

There grows an effortless *consecration* to the Divine who is sought after. And a necessary part of this consecration is self-purification. It is an inner purification : a relentless elimination of all that is contrary to the spirit of one's central endeavour, an abstention from contacts, physical, mental or vital, which tend to draw away from or contaminate in their results the purity of the seeking, a soulful tenderness and receptive expectancy which draws the Divine to reveal itself to the seeker.

All the faculties of the mind, its thought, will, imagination, are turned towards the Divine. The mind is gradually orientated towards the Divine on the wings of the heart's love. Once smitten with Love for the Supreme Beloved, the mind loses interest in the objects that held its attention before and turns to centre itself wholly round the Divine. Till that stage is reached, one may initially take the help of an Image or a Name to gather the energies of the mind and focus them on the Object of the seeking. Once the mind is trained to so concentrate itself, the image or the name gradually melts into the Reality, the Divine Personality they stand for and the consciousness of the seeker is engulfed in the Revelation. There is also the well-known process of hearing the glories of the Divine, *s´ravaṇam*, constant thinking of them and of Him whom they celebrate, *mananam*, and the settling of the mind on the Divine who is so adored, *dhyānam*. When this last condition deepens, the consciousness passes into an ecstatic trance, *samādhi*, in which the individual completely loses himself in the Object of his adoration.

Sri Aurobindo draws attention to the distinction between this Samadhi of the God-lover and the Samadhi of the discriminating Jnanin. The Bhakta's is an ecstatic experience, not the still and silent contemplation of the Jnanin of the Way of Knowledge. Here one does not pass into the Being of the Supreme but calls the Divine into oneself. Not peace of unity but bliss of union is the crown in the Way of Love.

Not only consecration of the mind but consecration of the body also. All outpourings of the will and energy are offered to the Divine. Here too there is a difference between the methods of dedication of the path of Bhakti and of the path of Works. In the latter it is the individual will that is taught to tune itself to the Higher Will of the Divine. The fulcrum is the will. But in the way of Devotion the motive-spring is love. Love is the dominant force which turns all action flowing towards the Divine as its dynamic outreaching. Work becomes at once a means for the expansion of love and a channel for the expression of love for the Divine in His manifold Becoming.

Thus does Bhakti, starting from whatever motive, gradually gather strength, shed its earthly dross and acquire the character of heavenly love which ever glows in the deepest centre of man, his psychic being. Sri Aurobindo enjoins upon the seeker to try and awaken this psychic element in himself so as to bring into operation its natural power of love which when it comes into its own, can alone by itself burn away the impediments and heal the imperfections in his nature. And Love has this supreme power, for in its pristine nature, it is the most divine dynamis in creation. It is, we may say, the yearning of the Divine in the individual form towards its Source, the Parent Divine Above. When the veils that cover it are removed and it is allowed to come to the front, there is no withstanding its imperious surge. From a spark it grows into a flame setting the whole being on fire for union with the Divine.

For the seeker of the Integral Yoga it is indeed not enough to realise this truth of love and union in his psychic depths alone. The union in love is to be realised in his other parts as well. They too have a secret aspiration and intention to participate in the bliss of union and contribute their characteristic powers in manifestation to add to the varied delight of the Union. The vital has a dynamic role to play; especially the higher vital with its large capacities for self-giving, heroism and mighty effectuations. The physical body too has its elements of stability and beauty to serve as a moving Temple of Love Divine.

Conclusion

THESE are broadly the three lines on which this Yoga can be pursued. Each one takes a particular faculty or power of the being for its base and fulcrum, and as the Yoga develops, that basic power is cultured and gradually raised to its highest potential. But in actual practice it is found that these different processes are not exclusive. Each one as it proceeds, touches and sets into motion the other processes also. Thus the doer of dedicated Works, serving the Lord with his will yoked to the supreme Will, finds a spontaneous welling up of devotion and love for Him on whom all his activities are centred. So also is the Bhakta moved to express his inner surrender and adoration of the Lord in the entire submission of his will to the Lord's and all his outer actions become movements of consecration. So again does the sadhaka of the way of Meditation and Knowledge find that his increasing awareness of the presence of the Divine everywhere fills him with an irresistible sense of wonder, devotion and surrender in which his dynamic will becomes a joyous slave of the Divine so perceived. It is not that these developments are successive to each other. They are more or less simultaneous.

The sadhaka of the Integral Yoga chooses that part of his being which is most developed and ready and starts with the mode of Yoga natural to it. Thus if he is preponderantly of a dynamic and expansive nature, he finds it natural to begin with his will disciplining itself in the way of Works; if he be primarily an emotional type and the heart is his central station of living he finds his way already selected for him; he takes the way of Love; or if he be more quietistic in temperament and accustomed to follow the lead of his mind, the *buddhi*, then the way of Meditation and Knowledge is the obvious line of progress for him. But human nature is not made of the mind alone or the heart alone or the will only; the being is complex and what moves one part or one power of it has its repercussions on the others in varying degrees. And especially in a Yoga like the Integral Yoga where the being in its entirety is exposed to the uplifting and transforming action of the Higher Shakti, it is most natural that alongside the main current of advance and progress, though in a lower key, other parts begin to respond in a contributory way and slowly gather strength to function on their own.

Whatever the starting-point and the main direction, the sadhana proceeds through four distinct phases. There is, first, a marked separation from the surface movements of the external nature and a growing awareness of a deeper and larger consciousness that makes itself felt. Thoughts, impulses, volitions begin to arise and function from this inner level of the being and the more one remains awake to this emerging expanse within the more is the normal human consciousness replaced by a deeper yogic consciousness. This new consciousness has to be brought into fuller sway, naturalised and made effective at all times.

As this is done with vigilance and patience, one tends to go still inward and discovers the real centre of life within, the soul or the psychic being, which is truly a portion of the Divine within oneself. The next phase in the sadhana is to draw this psychic element forward, evoke it in all the movements of mind, will and body, refer to it constantly, and thus organise one's whole life around the psychic. This operation is called the psychicisation of the being i.e., imparting the character of the psychic to all the rest of oneself, placing the whole of the being under the governance of the Psychic Monitor.

This gradual shift of the centre of one's consciousness from without to deep within has its repercussions in the opening of the higher levels of the being freed from the confines of the individual formulation. There is a natural extension of one's consciousness and a beginning of a living sense of unity with all in the universe around. One awakens to the throb in the universal Life of the same Divine Shakti that pulsates within oneself. This widening of the being goes on under the impulsion of the psychic *puruṣa* till the whole of the universe is embraced.

That is not all. There is an effortless move upward too. The consciousness in the mind either ascends to the regions above it or opens itself to the descent of what is above. These are the altitudes of the spiritual mind, the higher mind, the illumined mind, the intuitive mind etc., each of which has its own characteristic consciousness deriving from the Truth in manifestation, which is assimilated by the aspiring mind. There are several realisations of a transforming nature that the mind undergoes in its ascension. Thus for instance, above the boundaries of the Intellect, one is greeted by summits where all is silent : a Silence that impinges upon the consciousness as alone true and against the background of which all else appears temporary, fleeting and illusive. This is the belt of experience which has given rise to most of the theories of the illusoriness of the world and the sole reality of a Nihil, Nothing, an Ineffable. But that is not the final terminus.

Beyond the Silence are the glories of the *parārdha*, the Higher Worlds of Knowledge, Power and Joy with their corresponding principles and powers formulated in the individual. These are the planes of spiritual felicities which stir into life in the sadhaka. The vistas that open are endless, from plateau to plateau, say the seers of the Veda. Farthest known are the worlds of Sat, Chit and Ananda. They too can be realised, not merely in some Transcendent beyond the universe, but here in the individual they can be embodied and manifested. And ultimately that is the aim of this Creation. The immediate aim of the Yoga of Sri Aurobindo, however, is to rise above the bounds of the human mind, scale the heights of the higher, the illumined, the intuitive and still higher grades of the Mind and arrive at the Gnosis, the plane of Knowledge-Will which is the plenary manifestation of the Divine in its creative poise. That is the objective. The way to reach and receive it in one's own being and consciousness is the Yoga we have sketched out whose central process is best recapitulated in the words of Sri Aurobindo:

"A disclosure from within or a descent from above are the two sovereign ways of the Yoga-Siddhi. An effort of the external surface mind or emotions, a tapasya of some kind may seem to build up something of these things, but the results are usually uncertain and fragmentary, compared to the result of the two radical ways. That is why in this Yoga we insist always on an 'opening'—an opening inwards of the inner mind, vital, physical to the innermost part of us, the psychic, and an opening upwards to what is above the mind—as indispensable for the fruits of the sadhana.

"The underlying reason for this is that this little mind, vital and body which we call ourselves is only a surface movement and not our 'self' at all. ... The real Self is not anywhere on the surface but deep within and above. Within is the soul supporting an inner mind, inner vital, inner physical in which there is a capacity for universal wideness and with it for the things now asked for—direct contact with the truth of self and things, taste of a universal bliss, liberation from the imprisoned small-ness and sufferings of the gross physical body. . . . It is according to our psychology, connected with the small outer personality by certain centres of consciousness of which we become aware by Yoga. Only a little of the inner being escapes through these centres into the outer life, but that little is the best part of ourselves and responsible for our art, poetry, philosophy, ideals, religious aspirations, efforts at knowledge and perfection. But the inner centres are for the most part closed or asleep—to open them and make them awake and active is one aim of Yoga. As they open, the powers and possibilities of the inner being also are aroused in us, we awake first to a larger consciousness and then to a cosmic consciousness; we are no longer little separate personalities with limited lives but centres of a universal action and in direct contact with cosmic forces. Moreover, instead of being unwillingly play-things of the latter, as is the surface person, we can become to a certain extent conscious and masters of the play of nature—how far this goes depending on the development of the inner being and its opening upward to the higher spiritual levels. At the same time the opening of the heart centre releases the psychic being which proceeds to make us aware of the Divine within us and of the higher Truth above us.

"For the highest spiritual Self is not even behind our personality and bodily existence but is above it and altogether exceeds it. The highest of the inner centres is in the head, just as the deepest is the heart; but the centre which opens directly to the Self is above the head, altogether outside the physical body, in what is called the subtle body, *sūkṣma śarīra*. This Self has two aspects and the results of realising it correspond to these two aspects. One is static, a condition of wide peace, freedom, silence: the silent Self is unaffected by any action or experience; it impartially supports them but does not seem to originate them at all, rather to stand back detached or unconcerned, *udāsīna*. The other aspect is dynamic and that is experienced as a cosmic Self or Spirit which not only supports but originates and contains the whole cosmic action—not only that part of it which concerns our physical selves but also all that is beyond it—this world and all other worlds, the supraphysical as well as the physical ranges of the universe. Moreover, we feel the Self as one in all; but also we feel it as above all, transcendent, surpassing all individual birth or cosmic existence. To get into the universal Self—one in all—is to be liberated from ego; ego either becomes a small instrumental circumstance in the consciousness or even disappears from our consciousness altogether. This is the extinction or Nirvana of the ego. To get into the transcendent Self above all, makes us capable of transcending altogether even cosmic consciousness and action—it can be the way to that complete liberation from the world-existence which is called also extinction, *laya, mokṣa*, Nirvana.

"It must be noted however that the opening upward does not necessarily lead to peace, silence and Nirvana only. The sadhak becomes aware not only of a great, eventually an infinite peace, silence, wideness above us, above the head as it were and extending into all physical and supraphysical space, but also he can become aware of other things—a vast Force in which is all Power, a vast Light in which is all Knowledge, a vast Ananda in which is all bliss and rapture. At first they appear as something essential, indeterminate, absolute, simple, *kevala*: a Nirvana into any of these things seems possible. But we can come to see too that this Force contains all forces, this Light all lights, this Ananda all joy and bliss possible. And all this can descend into us. Any of them and all of them can come down, not peace alone; only the safest is to bring down first an absolute calm and peace, for that makes the descent of the rest more secure; otherwise it may be difficult for the external nature to contain or bear so much Force, Light, Knowledge or Ananda. All these things together make what we call the higher spiritual or Divine Consciousness. The psychic opening through the heart puts us primarily into connection with the individual Divine, the Divine in his inner relation with us; it is especially the source of love and bhakti. This upward opening puts us into direct relation with the whole Divine and can create in us the divine consciousness and a new birth or births of the spirit.

"When the Peace is established, this higher or Divine Force from above can descend and work in us. It descends usually first into the head and liberates the inner mind centres, then into the heart centre and liberates fully the psychic and emotional being, then into the navel and other vital centres and liberates the inner vital, then into the Muladhara and below and liberates the inner physical being. It works at the same time for perfection as well as liberation; it takes up the whole nature part by part and deals with it, rejecting what has to be rejected, sublimating what has to be sublimated, creating what has to be created. It integrates, harmonises, establishes a new rhythm in the nature. It can bring down too a higher nature until, if that be aim of the sadhana, it becomes possible to bring down the supramental forces and existence. All this is prepared, assisted, farthered by the work of the psychic being in the heart centre; the more it is open, in front, active, the quicker, safer, easier the working of the Force can be. The more love and bhakti and surrender grow in the heart, the more rapid and perfect becomes the evolution of the sadhana. For the descent and transformation imply at the same time an increasing contact and union with the Divine.

"This is the fundamental rationale of the sadhana. It will be evident that the two most important things here are the opening of the heart centre and the opening of the mind centres to all that is behind and above them. For the heart opens to the psychic being and the mind centres open to the higher consciousness and the nexus between the psychic being and the higher consciousness is the principal means of the siddhi. The first opening is effected by a concentration in the heart, a call to the Divine to manifest within us and through the psychic to take up and lead the whole nature. Aspiration, prayer, bhakti, love, surrender are the main supports of this part of the sadhana—accompanied by a rejection of all that stands in the way of what we aspire for. The second opening is effected by a concentration of the consciousness in the head (afterwards, above it) and an aspiration and call and a sustained will for the descent of the divine Peace, Power, Light, Knowledge, Ananda into the being—the Peace first or the Peace and Force together. Some indeed receive Light first or Ananda first or some sudden pouring down of Knowledge. With some there is first an opening which reveals to them a vast infinite Silence, Force, Light or Bliss above them and afterwards either they ascend to that or these things begin to descend into the lower nature. With others there is either the descent, first into the head, then down .to the heart level, then to the navel and below and through the whole body, or else an inexplicable opening— without any sense of descent—of peace, light, wideness or power, or else a horizontal opening into the cosmic consciousness or in a suddenly widened mind an outburst of knowledge. Whatever comes has to be welcomed—for there is no absolute rule for all—but if the peace has not come first, care must be taken not to swell oneself in exultation or lose the balance. The capital movement however is when the Divine force or Shakti, the power of the Mother comes down and takes hold, for then the organisation of the consciousness begins and the larger foundation of the Yoga."

Yoga Sadhana

A LETTER

1. It is not very necessary to study books on Advaita or Dvaita or Vishishtadvaita for practising Yoga. These philosophies have value as presentations of different spiritual experiences of the Reality in terms of the intellect. Each is valid, but from its own standpoint. Each is a view, but not the whole view of the Reality. This is seen when one ceases to merely theorise and speculate and proceeds to realise in experience. As you enter the inner domains of the soul or the higher reaches of the purified mind, the Reality, the Divine, reveals itself not in one aspect, not in one status of itself, but in many. You may start as a Dvaitin, as one approaching Another ; and the Divine may suddenly well up deep within you revealing itself as no other than your very own Self. Similarly, the Advaitin may be confronted with the presence of the Beloved around him claiming the adoration of the lover. The fact is the Divine has many aspects, many statuses and that is revealed to the seeker which is most natural to his inner being and most pertinent to his real need, whatever his mental preference.

So it is not at all indispensable that you should study the various philosophies for a successful pursuit of Yoga, though such a study rightly done, can help the mind to enlarge the bounds of its conceptual thinking and to appreciate the multiple character of spiritual experience in its approach to the many-sided Reality that is the Divine.

2. Regarding the experiences : each line of sadhana has its own kind of experiences leading to its definite realisation. The particular state which you describe as 'asamprajnata', where the difference between the seer and the seen fades away and the coiled up energy reaches the thousand-petalled lotus etc., is neither sought after nor normally experienced in the path of the Dvaitin. The Dvaitin would not be disposed to grant the same value to it as the Advaitin does.

Incidentally I may note in passing that 'flashes, blue spots, visions of gods, goddesses and great yogins' are not the only 'early mystical experiences'. These come by when there is an opening of the subtle vision. It may not happen for a long time or at all to many and yet they may well be firmly on the way. Their opening may be at different centres, heart, hearing, mind etc. and their experiences may be of the nature of an onsetting calm or peace, devotion, purity, clarity of knowledge, joy and so on.

3. The visions and experiences you describe are quite genuine. They indicate that you are awake on the subtler levels of existence where these things are usually active ; they also show that your being is ready to transcend the normal bounds of physical life and live on its higher ranges. Beyond this it is difficult to say. For each such vision, each experience, is to be weighed and valued in its own context, its background, its results in the waking consciousness. On these planes, there are many entities, benevolent, malevolent and other, and one cannot be too careful against likely masqueradings and enticing misdirections. One thing, however, is certain. If you have a central sincerity in your seeking, then whatever the initial stumblings and errors, the correct meaning and direction will come to you from within or without.

4. Pranayama is no part of the Integral Yoga of Sri Aurobindo though one may practise and use it for purposes of purifying and subtilising the mind, controlling the life-force etc. It can only be a means for a limited end which could well be achieved by less mechanical and more natural means in this Yoga. The period when Sri Aurobindo did Pranayama refers to his early days in Baroda when he practised the traditional Raja Yoga in part and had not yet come to formulate and develop the Yoga which was later built up by him after he came to Pondicherry and took up his spiritual mission exclusively.

5. Re. *Kuṇḍalinī Yoga* :

The signs of the awakening of the Kundalini are unmistakable. There is considerable heat in the body, especially in the region of the Muladhara. Those whose subtle audition is sensitive are said to hear a low droning sound like the murmur of bees when the Kundalini is set active.

When the Kundalini passes through any centre or chakra in its upward ascent, there is a particular experience of bliss at that centre. It is concretely felt and one can know which particular centre has been touched and negotiated. Also one gains a control or the beginnings of a mastery over the *tattva* or principle governed by that centre.

6. Thus far regarding the various queries you have made. Now coming to the most important point in your letter as to what path you should adopt and what discipline you may best follow, the answer is it depends upon your goal in life. And while setting a goal for yourself, it goes without saying that you take into account the equipment with which you are endowed, the nature of your temperament and being, the kind of *saṁskāras* to which your mind is habituated. It is obvious you are not satisfied with the normal type of physical life common in the world. Then, is it a kind of sattvic life governed by the light of the mind and warmth of the soul that you seek ? Or is it a definite turn to the life spiritual ? And if it is a spiritual

career that you choose, do you seek only the salvation of the soul, mukti, or a liberation of the whole of your being,—the soul, mind, life and body,—from the hold of Ignorance, and its all-round growth and fulfilment in the Divine Consciousness with its essential powers of Knowledge, Will and Joy? If it is the former, any of the traditional lines of Yoga may be followed. If the latter then the Integral, Poorna, Yoga of Sri Aurobindo is the obvious choice.

You ask what is the practical method of this Yoga. Put broadly, the Yoga begins with a keen aspiration for the Truth of life, for the Divine. It proceeds through a willed opening in the heart, in the mind and in all the rest of the being to the Higher Consciousness of the Divine; a rejection of all that is contrary to the Object of one's seeking; and a progressive surrender, placing of oneself in the hands of the Yoga Shakti, the Divine Power which can be directly received and experienced through the Grace of the Guru acting through a look, a word — spoken or written — or in other innumerable ways. This call and opening of oneself in consciousness to the Divine Shakti and the responsive incoming or unveiling of the Power work out the process of this Yoga which proceeds in three main movements viz., first, the realisation of the Divine within oneself; second, the realisation and identification with the Divine extended in the cosmos; and third, a transformation of nature leading to a self-transcendence into the plenary status of Vijnana, the Gnosis.

Thus it will be seen that this discipline is largely psychological to begin with; it acquires a spiritual character as it progresses. Physical and psycho-physical means adopted in other lines of Yoga could be used here also as feeders to the main process.

You refer to Sri Aurobindo's remark that this yoga is the easiest. That is indeed so because it is the most natural of all yogas inasmuch as it only concentrates the methods and accelerates the process of Nature in evolution. To grow, to expand and arrive at an acme of perfection which rejects no main element that has been evolved but raises each to its fullest value is the one aim that Nature pursues in all the million forms of her making and through her thousandfold processes. The aim of Sri Aurobindo's Yoga is the same. Only it is not content to let things develop in the slow, leisurely motion of the universal Nature. It takes up the fundamental operation of that Nature, applies it with a firm and conscious direction in the awakened being of man and seeks to precipitate within a single life-time results that would otherwise takes ages to appear.

Sadhana and the Body

Sri Aurobindo has written : ' Sadhana has to be done in the body, it cannot be done by the soul without the body'. Would it not be easier to do the sadhana when one is relieved of the gross material body and lives in the subtle body alone?

Sadhana cannot be done except with the physical body. The Earth, the Physical is the field of progress, sadhana, evolution. Even the Gods, it is said in the Scriptures, have to come down on the earth, take a physical body and do tapasya if they want to enlarge or exceed themselves. There is no movement of progress on planes other than the physical. Over there things are all set to type and those worlds are content in their typal perfection.

Once you leave the body, the part nearest to the physical, the subtle-physical rushes to find some shelter in some physical abode, in the environs of the family or friends, in trees etc. The rest of the being, the mental and the vital parts clinging to the psychic entity within pass through the intervening planes or stages to the psychic world where the central being rests for recuperation and rest till the time is come for the next incarnation. It does not do sadhana. It simply rests and silently prepares for the coming birth.

Of course there are cases, very very rare though, of persons who after passing away have continued to *live* in the earth-atmosphere, for shorter or longer periods, and exert themselves for the good of those on earth. But they have done so not for sadhana but to make available to all the fruits of their sadhana done during their *life-time on earth, in the physical body.*

The physical ensures a stability, a containing continuity which the other strata of the being cannot provide so naturally to the workings of the Spirit.

Divine Grace and Human Effort

If ultimately one has to depend upon the Divine Grace, what is the necessity of personal effort by meditation, concentration etc.?

It is true that the Divine Grace is finally the deciding factor. It is quite impossible in spiritual life to effect certain decisive results by human effort alone. It is the intervention and operation of the Grace that precipitates the steps at crucial stages. But there are two sides to this working of the Divine Grace. The manifestation of the Grace is usually preceded by a *state of grace* in the sadhaka. And this state is the slow result of a long preparation and tapasya, whether known to the surface personality of man or not known. Even when the impact of the Grace appears to be sudden we can be sure that there has been ample preparation behind it, either in the present life or in the past.

Not only the manifestation but the working of Grace also has to be supported by human effort. As Sri Aurobindo says, the Divine Grace will act only in the conditions of Truth. The recipient has at every moment to put himself on the side of Truth and reject every element of Un-truth that is foreign to the presence of the Grace. This demands a ceaseless discipline of aspiration, rejection, surrender. The central sincerity has to be spread to all the different parts of the being so as to build a temple of oneself to receive and contain the Divine Grace. Otherwise the Grace recedes.

So human effort is indispensable both prior to the advent and subsequent to the manifestation of the Grace. Tapasya is necessary to invoke the Higher Power. Sadhana is required to receive and keep the gifts of the Grace. Till the higher working is securely established and the charge of the completely consecrated being is taken up by the Divine Shakti, personal effort is essential. The Grace works more rapidly and victoriously in such a responsive and dynamic *ādhāra* than in one given to tamasic resignation and indolence.

Inner Strength and Will-Power

What is the difference between Inner Strength and Will-Power? How to generate and strengthen the Will-Power?

Inner strength refers to the development of the *inner* being of man as distinct from his surface personality which is all he is normally aware of. This inner being consisting of the inner mind, inner vital and the subtle-physical organised round the central being or the soul, carries with it the essence of its evolutionary labour which is reflected in the state of its development, its strength and power as an individual manifestation of the Spirit. This state of the inner being is not dependent on outer circumstances, it exists by itself supporting the further evolution of the soul through the frontal personality. It may or may not be reflected in its fullness in the outer nature which is chosen to suit the purpose for which the particular birth has been taken.

This inner strength, being a developed power of the soul in manifestation, can be increased by the cultivation of higher soul-values and their practice. When so done the inner strength not only gets added nourishment but it comes forward to overtly support and participate in the growth of the evolving person. Otherwise it lies as a reserve behind the activity of the surface elements.

What is normally called will-power is clearly different from this strength. It is a projection in nature of the soul's power for effectuation. Will is the focus of the demand of the being to exist, to live and increase. It is there in the mind, in the life-force, even in the physical body. In some it takes distinct shape and dominates and moulds life as it desires. In others it is incipient and weak, has no power to assert itself, goes under at every opposition and man becomes just a creature of circumstances. But it is possible to build it up into a force for growth and mastery. It has to be cultivated in the way the muscles of the body are developed. One has to activate the will, exercise it deliberately and gradually increase its sway and power. It is easy to sense one's will-element in the mind i.e., in a thought or idea that arises in the mind. If it is a healthy idea, one must make it an occasion to exercise the will and develop it. Pursue the idea, exert yourself to translate it into action. There are likely to be obstructions; but do not give up at the first hurdle. Strive, get over it and proceed to work out the idea. That way the will develops and grows. Similarly if there be a wrong thought or idea, resist the temptation to yield to it. In the very process of thus opposing a movement contrary to the growth of the being, the will acquires a strength and you will have gained a larger and stronger fund of will-power for the next trial of strength. The same holds good on all the levels of the being, the spiritual, the emotional, the nervous and the physical. Every circumstance that presents itself can be utilised for the exercise and growth of the will-power and consequent development of one's individuality.

As the discipline proceeds, the inner strength begins to come forward from its depths and express itself more and more overtly in this will-power which, ultimately, after its dross of desire and egoism is burnt away in the fire of tapasya, transforms itself into a pure dynamis of the soul.

Law of Karma

You have stated[1] that the powerful man who exerts himself prospers whatever his moral deserts whereas his virtuous competitor lacking the requisite will-power fails to make good. Why is it so?

This statement has been made while discussing the Law of Karma and its manifold working. Karma means that a given output of energy calls back the same energy in the form of a result. The energy that flows back is commensurate with the quality and the quantity of the output. The nature of what is put forth decides the nature of what comes in consequence. Thus if a certain effort is made in the moral direction the result too will be on the moral plane. A moral discipline for instance will promote a moral strength and increase the moral courage. Its results are not to be sought for in material terms. For results in the material sphere, exertion has got to be on the material level. Thus a moral effort will produce a moral effect, a spiritual effort produce a spiritual result and an output of force in the physical economy of things

[1] *Sri Aurobindo : Studies in the Light of His Thought*, p. 54.

produce results in a physical way. This in brief is the doctrine of Karma in pure theory. In practice, however, the fact that man lives and acts simultaneously on several planes of existence introduces a complicating factor of the interaction of their several movements. There is also the factor of the Karma of the environment, the Karma or heredity etc. But to return to the question.

It is clear why success or failure in the material field is not dependent on the moral qualifications of a man. It depends mainly on the energies poured out in the material way, the labour that goes into the physical working. Goodness or badness of the doer has little to do with the matter. For moral excellence there is a moral consequence, not material advancement. Each line of Karma is different from the other and an output in one should not be confused with results in another flowing from a cause in their own kind.

Meditation

I begin to get thoughts in the mind the moment I sit for meditation. However much I may try they do not stop and even after half an hour of effort I do not get more than a minute of peace and quiet. There is an exhaustion at the end. How long should the exertion be made? How to quiet the mind?

It is not that thoughts begin to come in when one meditates. Thoughts are there all the time, only one does not normally take notice of them as one is occupied with something or the other. When one begins to meditate, all the mental faculties are withdrawn from outer activities and one gets aware of the movement of thoughts some of which come from outside and some appear to rise from within. To struggle with them and sit upon them is not always the best method. Keeping a central remembrance of the purpose for which one is sitting, one can let the thoughts run their course; only one must keep to the remembrance taking care not to run with the thoughts. One does not succeed immediately, but there should be a patient and persistent come-back to the main Thought every time there is

7

a sliding into the running current of thought-activity. In course of time the thoughts dwindle.

Another method is to put a will and concentrate or gather the consciousness round the object of meditation ignoring the existence of other thoughts. Aids like Japa or visualisation of an image or a felt invocation to the Divine Person who embodies the object of your seeking, may be used to draw the mind from its running course and still the thought-movement. If you cannot centre the mind around the object of meditation immediately, keep it centred in a circle closely related to that object. Foreign movements will automatically recede for want of supporting attention.

In any case there should be no strain. To learn to relax and release the consciousness in a flow on the object of seeking is the secret of meditation. Reading of elevating literature, recitation of a few rhythmic passages from scriptures for a little while, create a helpful background for meditation.

It is hard to quiet the mind by one's own effort. The easier way is to remember and conceive of a Silence, a Quiet that is there behind everything, behind your mind, and call upon the Silence to enter into you. If done with faith there is bound to be a response, sooner or later, and then you have only to let yourself into the folds of the Quiet or the Silence that comes in an enveloping movement.

Disturbing Thoughts

Whenever anyone known to me is reported to be ill or starts out on a journey, I get inauspicious thoughts. What is to be done on such occasions?

Usually it is attachment or some kind of self-interest that gives rise to such apprehensions, *atisnehah pāpas'anki.* At the root of such movement is a fear on the part of the ego that it may lose a support. It may also be that such thoughts and fears are drawn to itself by a nature or a mind which is habitually morbid and constantly dwells on the wrong side of things. There are, in the present constitution of the universe, a number of beings and forces which embody dark movements like anxiety, fear, terror etc. and they are always on the look out for likely receptacles for their activities. The only way to counter their invasion is to resolutely shut them out, refuse to look at them much less entertain them. It is difficult but it has to be done in some form or the other. This is a negative way of rejection. The positive way is to place reliance on the Divine and every time such thoughts and fears come in, to refer them or surrender them to the Divine and yourself remain trustfully quiet. After all nobody is going to be helped by your entertaining these apprehensions. If at all, by giving a mental body to these amorphous ideas you help them in their attempt to effectuate themselves and thus cause indirect injury to those for whom you profess concern. On the other hand if you remember the Divine on such occasions there is a double advantage : the wrong suggestions melt away before the Light which you invoke and you do not give them a chance to formulate themselves in shape : a helpful vibration is set going for the benefit of the person concerned.

Sadhana and Apparel

I have a liking for bright colours in clothes. As a sadhika, is it desirable for me to avoid wearing such clothes as they may attract other people's attention which might affect my consciousness? Should I cease taking interest in such dresses?

There is nothing at all wrong or unspiritual in wearing bright or beautiful clothes. Beauty is an important part of the Divine Manifestation and it is a kind of perverse denial to refuse to participate in that movement. As much as Knowledge, Power and Joy, Beauty also—with all its picturesque variety—is a facet of God to be manifested in each individual, even as it is abundantly manifest in Nature on all the planes of existence.

The question about attracting other people's attention is a little more complicated. There it is really a matter which depends upon oneself. If there is no intention of drawing attention from outside, in however concealed a form, then, as a rule no such attention is drawn. Whatever attention may be directed from others would not be of such a nature as to produce vibrations of consequence in your consciousness. It is usually when something in you wants and waits for it that there is an impact of that kind. It does not matter what you wear or do not wear. But it does matter why you wear it. To look pretty or beautiful is not unspiritual or immoral. But to embellish oneself in order to provoke admiration or invite attention, consciously or subconsciously, is not very wholesome for one's well-being.

Sadhana and Gifts

Can a sadhak accept gifts from others? Will there not be an exchange of undesirable vital forces? What should a sadhak do if forced to accept gifts by relatives?

Naturally, a gift always carries with it something of the person who gives it. It may be goodwill, affection, sentiment of regard or devotion. It may also be a claim subtly laid on the recipient. At its worst it can be a physical means to establish a relation with the receiver for any purpose, nefarious or otherwise.

It follows that it is the spirit accompanying the present that should determine the right course —to accept or not to accept. In ordinary social life it is indeed difficult to refuse gifts from friends, relatives etc. And the obligation that ensues on accepting a present is usually offset by a return-present in due time. Where however, the recipient is not in a position to return, the obligation remains ; a vital claim is established and his freedom of movement in his relations with the giver is compromised to that extent. In spiritual life, luckily, it is not incumbent on the sadhaka to conform to this social convention of gifts. He can impose on himself a wholesome discipline of not accepting any presents at all; or if he is obliged to accept by special circumstances, he should inwardly offer it to the Divine within and accept on His behalf. Thereby he saves himself from the consequences of the gift.

Sadhana in the Ashram

It is said that in the past sadhaks had had several experiences in their sadhana which they do not get these days. Why? Is it that the method of working of the Mother has changed? Or is it a necessary stage in the collective sadhana?

In a collective life like the Ashram, there are certain dominant factors which stamp themselves on the consciousness of the constituting members. The most important of these is the working of the Yoga-Shakti of Sri Aurobindo and the Mother. The central feature of its workings is always reflected in the inner life of the inmates whether all are conscious of it or not. That is why during the earlier years when the Mother was working upon the mental and vital planes subjecting them to the pressure of the descending Power, sadhaks here used to experience so much activity in the inner layers of their mind and vitality. Visions, voices, inrushes of knowledge, power, joy—all these experiences were the indices of the stir of the general movement in the mental and vital layers of the collectivity. As the work was completed, as far as could be, on these planes, the emphasis was shifted to the subtle-physical and physical planes and for the past one decade or more, the Mother has been directing the Yoga-Force on the physical and below the physical. These layers are denser than those of mind or life regions and naturally the results of the pressure thereon take time to express themselves in the *ādhāras* of individuals, especially if they are not particularly attentive and responsive.

Comparatively speaking, the response was readier and more spectacular in the mental and the vital parts of the collective being for the reason that they are subtler by nature and nearer the spirit in the gradation of Existence. Besides, the aspiration and preparation of the sadhaks was more adequate in these parts than it has been in the physical. Even so, it is not that there are no experiences now. Experiences there are, only they are not of the kind people were used to. Those who are sensitive do see the results of the impact of the Higher Force and Consciousness on the physical system, specially the stronger resistance of the body to the forces of disintegration, greater resilience in responding to touches of the Mother's Force and so on.

Movements Outside and the Ashram

There are spiritual movements (like that of Unity people in Missouri) which often speak and preach and believe in what the Mother believes, believe in some sort of a new and better world for which the time is now ripe, and emphasise on the spiritual meaning of religion; their whole approach to all personal and other problems is spiritual. But they are not consciously in touch with the Mother. No doubt it must be the New Force that is at work. But would it make any difference to them if they turned consciously towards the Mother? I mean in the process of their transformation, in the realisation etc.

When new truths begin to descend into the earth atmosphere there are many who receive them. But each grasps and formulates according to the nature and competence of the mind that perceives. Some receive them fragmentarily, some in a fuller measure. It is only the rare few, in fact those who can be said to be born to embody and manifest these truths, that see them whole and express them adequately. Now, the Ideal of a perfect life on earth, the vision of a New Age of God-men has been there for a long time and it has been glimpsed and promulgated in inspired utterances by several men in several communities and various efforts have been made to translate them in actual life. But rarely have any two such movements been identical. Their language may appear to be very much the same but there is always a difference in their import and their application.

Coming to the matter in question, though there are today a number of movements aiming to prepare and equip for a new life of harmony, peace and unity, their objectives, methods and their whole outlook on life are radically different from those of the Teaching and Yoga of Sri Aurobindo and the Mother. 'Spiritual movements', like the one you speak of, have the betterment of the human lot as their aim. Reduction of stress and strain, amelioration of conditions, increasing happiness and security in life are what they generally have in view. To this end they draw upon or adapt the tenets of one religion or another or formulate some sort of a system combining the fundamentals of all religions with an element of occult practice. But our endeavour is set in a totally different key. We do Yoga not for human ends, however laudable, but for a Divine Purpose and this Purpose includes a radical, not piecemeal, change of the human nature into its ultimate term of super-nature—a real transformation of the whole of the living man which is not envisaged elsewhere. The Divine has willed that a higher Consciousness shall manifest and lift up the entire life in creation to a new dimension. The Mother embodies the Power that works the Will and She has chosen some from humanity who are prepared to surrender themselves to the Call of the Divine and make themselves its instruments for the reception, manifestation and establishment of the New Consciousness.

Naturally though the immediate field of the Mother's direction of the New Consciousness-Force that is now manifesting, its physical centre, is the Ashram community, the range of its influence is wider and in course of time the whole earth will come under its Glory. Meanwhile—till this divine Power of Knowledge-Will gets into its full stride and begins to function on an organised basis—all progressive movements working for the elevation of man, for the clearance of the backwaters of Ignorance, darkness and misery, receive and will continue to receive an indirect help and impetus from the Force centrally acting through the person of the Mother. It goes without saying that if any individual or movement turned directly to Her and received inspiration and guidance immediately from Her that would make a tremendous difference. It does make a difference whether you stand directly below a shower or are content to receive the distant spray.

Gayatri

There is a popular belief that the Sri Gayatri mantra is not very responsive to the spiritual aspirant in this Yuga. But I am attracted by that Mantra and have been doing its japa. I am of the view that the Light that is invoked in the Gayatri Mantra is the supramental Light and the aim is supramentalisation. Is that correct?

I am not aware of any such popular belief regarding the incompatibility of the Gayatri with spiritual life in this age or any other. On the other hand in almost all upāsanās, Vaidic as well as Tantric, there is a Gayatri addressed to the Devata that is adored. Possibly the claim made in the *stutipāṭhas* (laudatory stanzas) of the Mantra that it promotes all the four traditional aims of life, *dharma, artha, kāma* and *mokṣa,* may have given rise to the belief that since other interests also are served by the Mantra it is to that extent inimical to true spiritual ends.

In these matters it is as a rule safe to welcome a Mantra for which one feels some attraction, on practising which one feels happy. It is a friendly Mantra which has affinity with something in you.

I am not sure that the aim of the Gayatri is supramentalisation; I rather think it is not. This much is certain : the Sun that is addressed is not the solar orb in the sky but the Sun of Spiritual Truth at the head of creation whose symbol in this universe is the physical sun. The Light that flows from that Sun is the illumined energy of the creative Consciousness that is massed therein. The Vaidic Gayatri (of Rishi Vishwamitra) prays for the activation of one's intelligence by the rays of that Light. A spiritual illumination of the mind, the highest evolved part of man is what is sought for. And this is indispensable in all spiritual disciplines that proceed through an awakening and growth in the Way of Jnana, Knowledge of the Divine, though it may not be very relevant for the Way of Bhakti.

Supramentalisation is far different and much more. It implies the lighting up of not only the mind but the whole of one's being, not merely rendering it luminous with knowledge but charging it in other ways of being also viz., feeling, will, action etc. so as to transform the human nature into the Divine. That is the aim of Sri Aurobindo's Gayatri which runs :

Tat savitur varam rūpam jyotiḥ parasya dhīmahi, yannaḥ satyena dīpayet.

Let us meditate on the most auspicious (best) form of Savitri, on the Light of the Supreme which shall illumine us with the Truth.